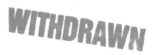

# A DENTIST'S TOOLS

# A DENTIST'S TOOLS

## KENNY DeSANTIS

Photographs by
## PATRICIA A. AGRE

*Introduction by Bruce E. Golden, D.D.S.*

G. P. PUTNAM'S SONS • New York

# ACKNOWLEDGMENTS

Special thanks to Dr. Steven Moss, Chairman and Professor, Department of Pediatric Dentistry, New York University College of Dentistry, New York City, NY; Michael J. Vitale, D.M.D., Bronxville, NY; Eugene Humbert, D.D.S., Family Dental Service of the Family Health Center, White Plains Hospital Medical Center, White Plains, NY; William Hurwitz, D.D.S., New York City, NY; Dr. Walner Almada de Oliveira, Franca, São Paulo, Brazil; Agnes Villeneuve, Dental Assistant, Hudson, P.Q., Canada; Morty Baker, D.D.S., Hudson, P.Q., Canada; Ellen Smith; Hazel Ross; Nancy Giacci; Jennifer Sklias; Simone Murray; and Carol Moscinski.

A most special thank you to the White Plains, NY, office of Bruce E. Golden, D.D.S.; Lisa A. Ritter, D.M.D.; Catherine Mingone, R.H.; Terry Thompson, Dental Assistant; Aurea Salas, Dental Assistant; Wendy St. Val, Receptionist; Peppi Nitta, Dental Assistant; and all the little people who have benefited from their expert and gentle ministrations.

There is an increasing trend for dentists to supply office personnel with protective gloves, masks, and eyewear so as to adhere to office hygiene procedures described in the infection control guidelines recommended by the Center for Disease Control (CDC) and the American Dental Association (ADA).

Library of Congress Cataloging-in-Publication Data
DeSantis, Kenny. A dentist's tools. Summary: Introduces the tools a dentist uses to inspect, clean,
polish, and repair teeth. 1. Dentistry–Juvenile
literature. 2. Children–Preparation for dental
care–Juvenile literature. [1. Dentistry. 2. Dental care]
I. Agre, Patricia, ill. II. Title. [RK63.D47 1988b]
617.6′0028 89-8375
ISBN 0-399-61231-9

10 9 8 7 6 5 4 3 2

*To*
*Bruce Golden,*
*Lisa Ritter,*
*Catherine Mingone,*
*Wendy St. Val,*
*Aurea Salas,*
*Peppi Nitta,*
*Terry Thompson*

For many generations dentists have struggled to decrease the pain and anxiety suffered by their patients. Yet, for too many people in every age group, an impending dental appointment induces apprehension or even dread. Dental instruments and their lay terms—drill, needle, pick—may provoke intense fear.

As a teacher and practitioner of pediatric dentistry, I utilize a method of "behavior shaping" which is founded upon honesty and openness with children. My own teacher, Professor Harold Kane Addelston, taught me to tell and show children exactly what I am going to do. I then proceed with my treatment while encouraging the child to watch in a small mirror. The real value of this open and intellectual method of anxiety management has been to eliminate the fear of the "unknown."

Every day of my professional life reinforces my positive feeling for this approach, for I not only see children's dental health improve, I also see their self-esteem take a growth step. It is refreshing to see children proud of their successful dental visit.

It is my happy fortune that the author and photographer have provided an honest look at the art and science of dentistry from the child-patient's eye level. I am sure it will serve children, parents, and dentists.

**Bruce E. Golden, D.D.S.**
*Diplomate, American Board of Pediatric Dentistry*
*Clinical Associate Professor,*
*New York University, College of Dentistry*

There are many tools in a dentist's office. They are called instruments. These instruments help the dentist take care of your teeth.

Some dentists work with hygienists. A hygienist's job is to make sure your teeth are clean. Instruments help the hygienist too.

You may have a lot of questions about a visit to the dentist. You may want to know about the different tools—"What is that?" "What's it for?" "How will it feel?"

We hope this book will help to answer some of those questions.

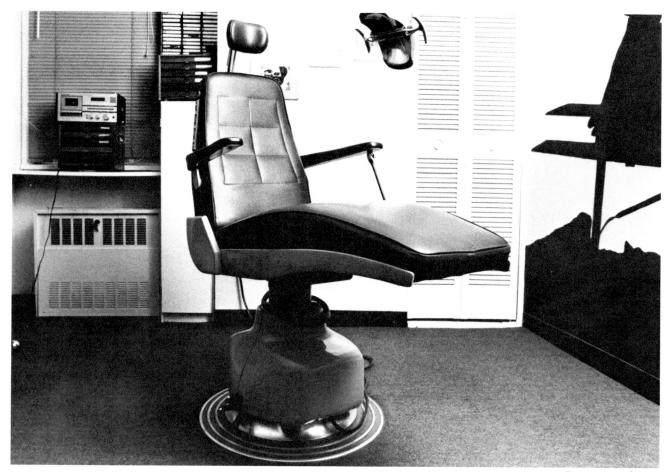

Dentist's chair

## CHECKUP
When you visit the dentist, he will look at your teeth to see if they are healthy. This is called a checkup.

You will be asked to sit in the **dentist's chair.** This chair can be fixed so that it is just right for someone your size. It can be moved up

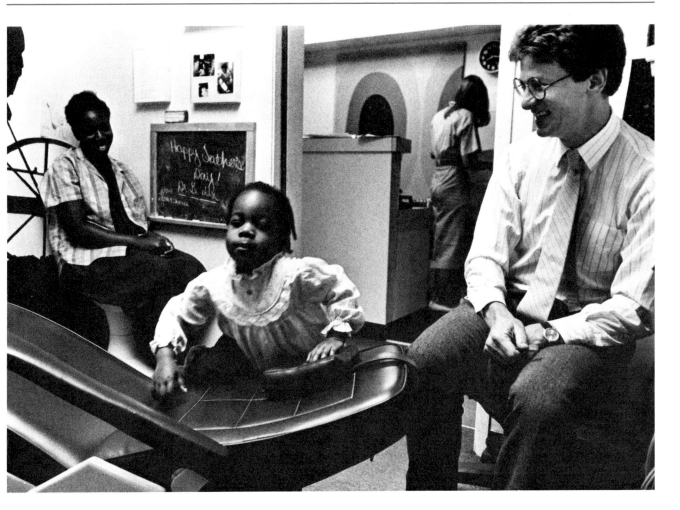

and down and tipped forwards and
backwards. If you ask, the dentist
may give you a ride.

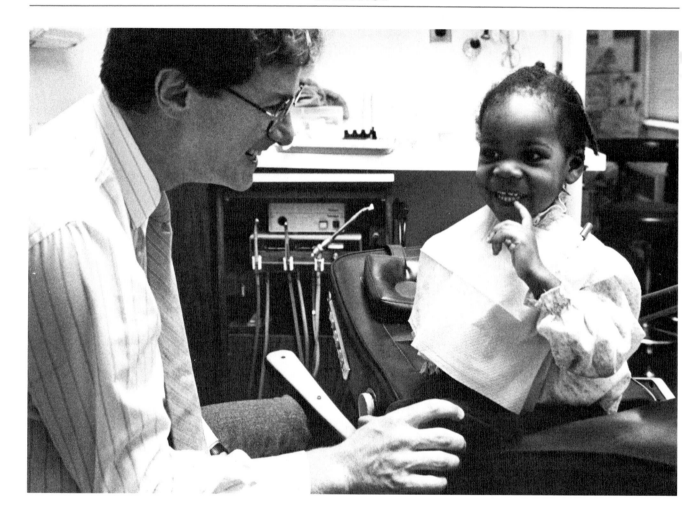

Before checking your teeth, the
dentist clips a paper **bib** around your
neck. It will keep your shirt or
blouse clean.

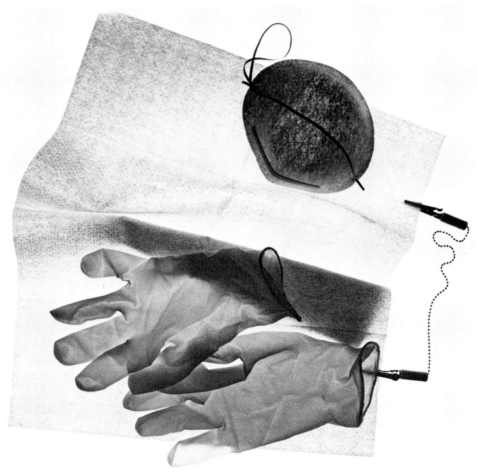

Bib, mask, gloves

Most dentists wear **rubber gloves** and some wear **masks.** They do this to protect you from germs.

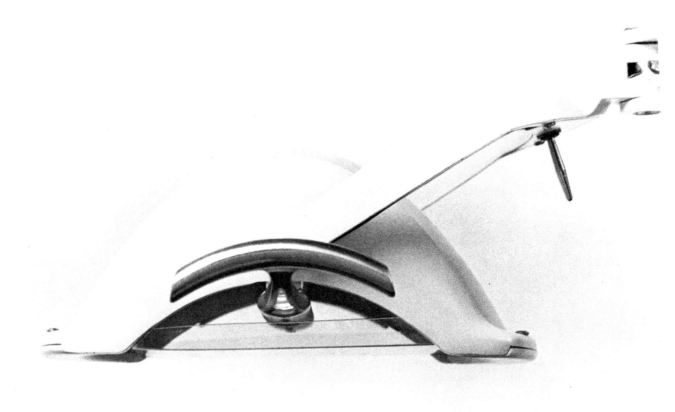

Light

Once you are settled in the chair, the dentist turns on a bright **light.** This light helps him to see inside your mouth. Nearby is a small tray. It holds some of the tools that are used to check your teeth.

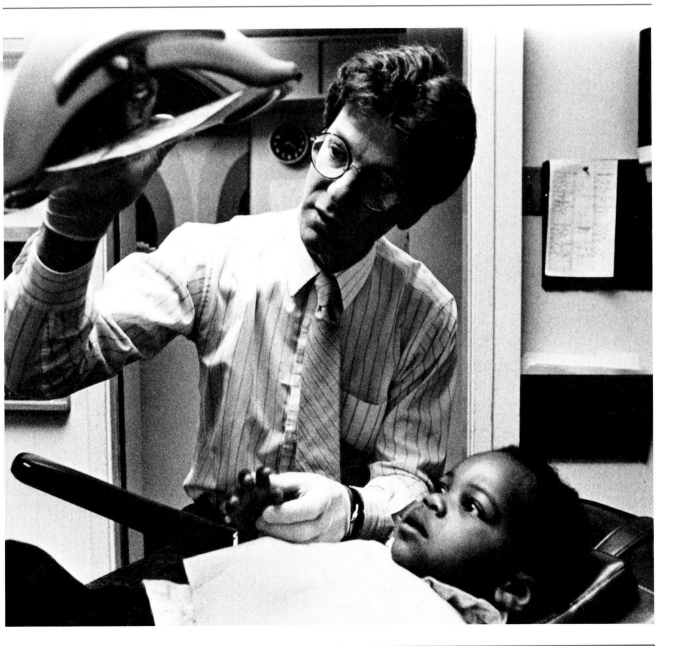

On the tray there is a **mouth mirror** and an **explorer.** The mouth mirror is used to look at your teeth. By moving it gently from tooth to tooth, the dentist can see if they look the way they should. He uses the explorer to feel the top and sides of each tooth to see if they are hard and smooth. You can tell when the dentist finds a soft or rough spot because the tip of the explorer gets caught and you can feel a little tug. The dentist also uses the explorer to count your teeth.

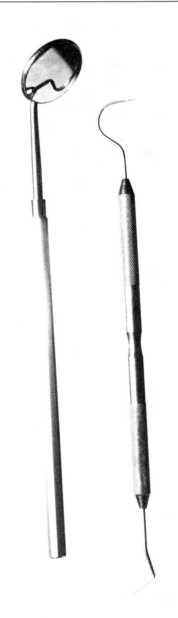

Mouth mirror and explorer

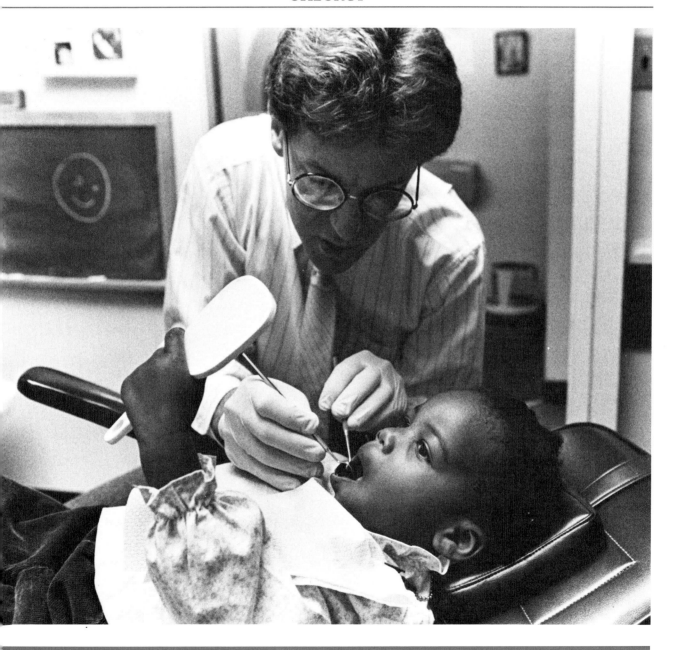

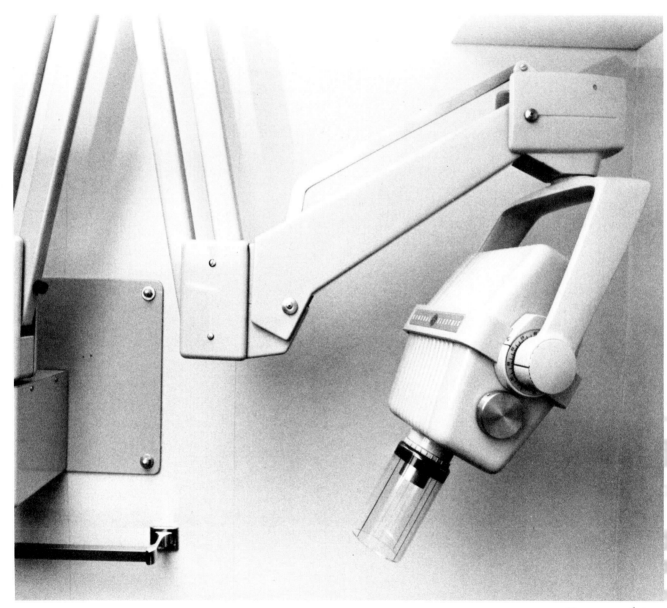

X-ray machine

To see underneath, inside, and in between your teeth, the dentist may want to take some X-ray pictures. To do this an **X-ray machine** is used. This is a special kind of camera. It is snuggled up close to your face, but it doesn't touch you.

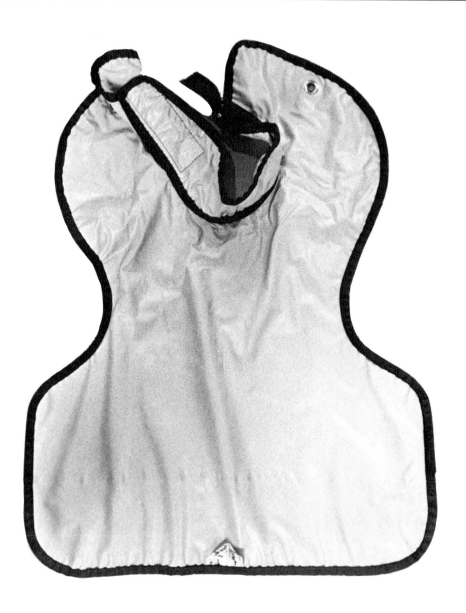

Lead apron

To make sure that only your teeth are X-rayed, your neck and chest are covered with a **lead apron.** It will feel heavy.

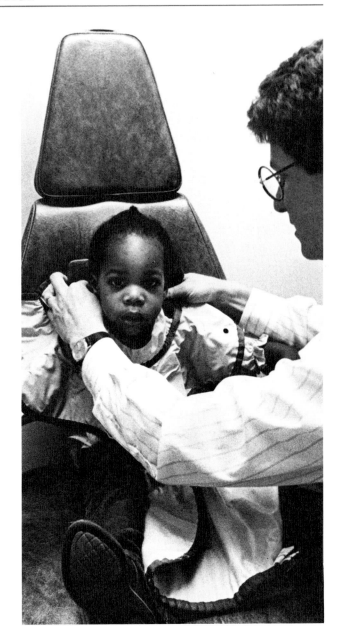

X-ray film goes in your mouth, not in the camera. To get pictures of your front teeth, the film is held in place with your thumb or your teeth. For pictures of your back teeth, you bite down on a cardboard or plastic film holder called a **bite-wing tab.**

Taking an X-ray takes a few seconds. For that short time, you will be asked to hold as still as a statue. When you hear a hum, a click, or a buzz, you will know the X-ray has been taken. Very soon the dentist will take the film out of your mouth and the apron off your chest.

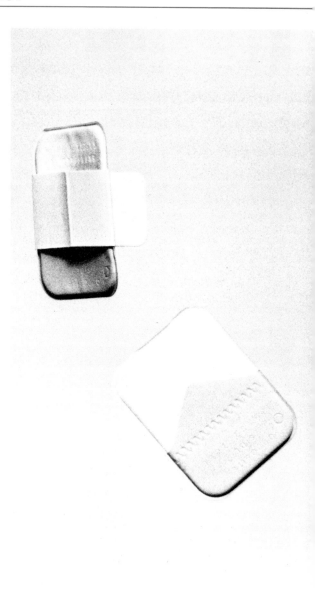

X-ray film and bitewing tab

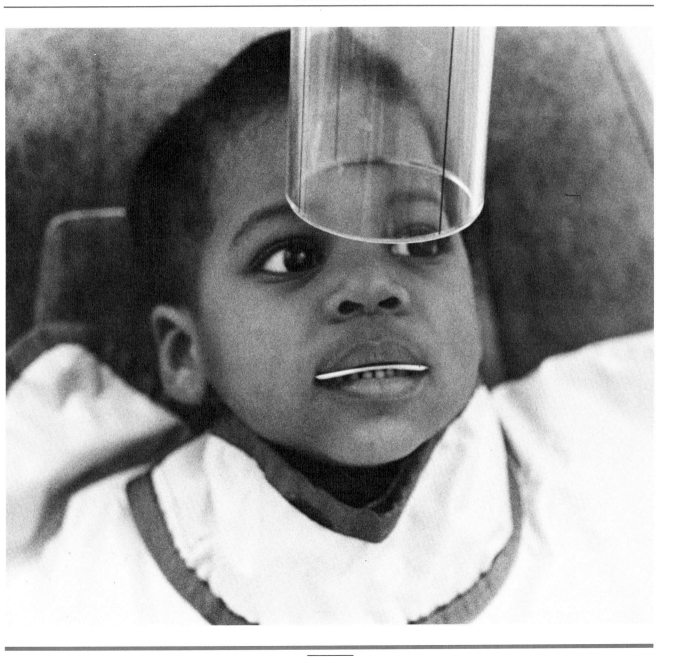

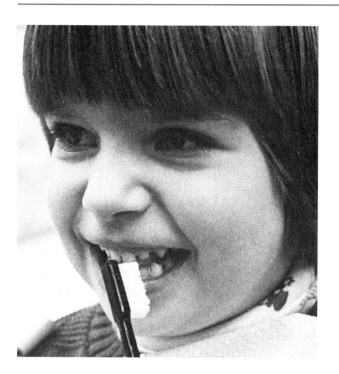

## PREVENTION

### Cleaning, Polishing, Protecting

The most important thing you can do to keep your teeth strong and healthy is to make sure they are clean. Clean teeth have no plaque on them. Plaque is a sticky layer of germs. It is bad for your teeth because it can make them decay.

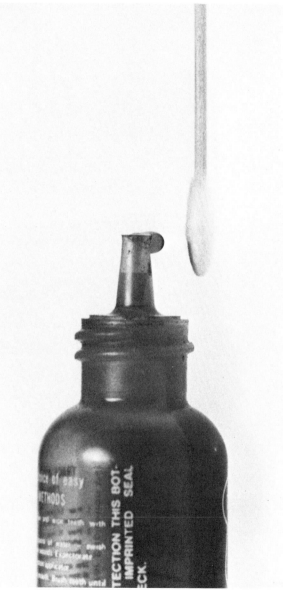

Disclosing solution

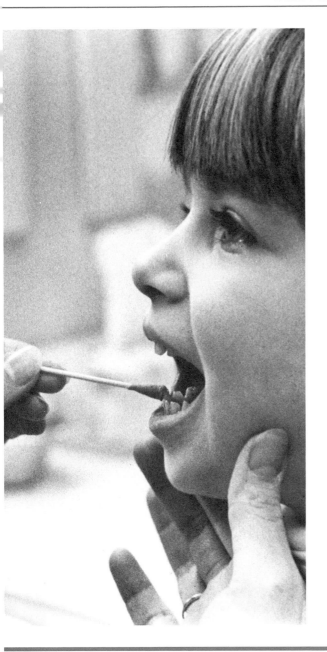

The best way to get rid of plaque is to brush and floss your teeth carefully every day. The hygienist shows you how to do this.

First, you are asked to brush your teeth, all by yourself. Then the hygienist checks to see how clean you got them by painting them bright red with cherry- or strawberry-flavored **disclosing solution.** (Sometimes you chew on a disclosing tablet). After swishing out your mouth with water, you will be surprised when you look in the mirror! All the places you brushed clean will be white. All the places you missed will still be red.

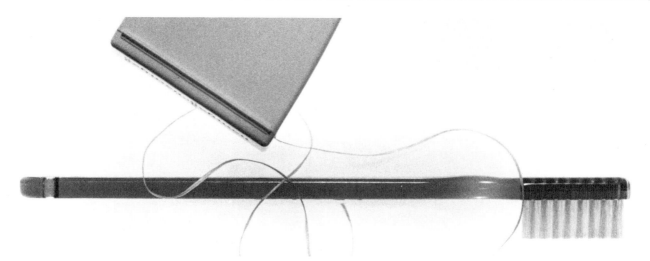

Toothbrush and dental floss

It's hard to do a good job of cleaning your teeth when you are little. That's why the hygienist teaches your mom or dad how to brush and floss for you. The **toothbrush** cleans the tops and sides of your teeth. **Dental floss** cleans in between them. If there is **tartar** on your teeth, the hygienist will gently scrape it off with a **scaler.** Tartar is plaque and minerals that have gotten too hard to brush away.

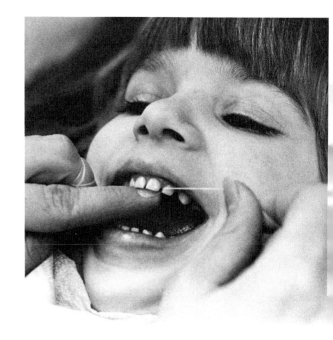

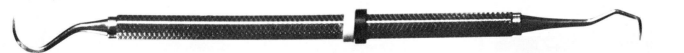

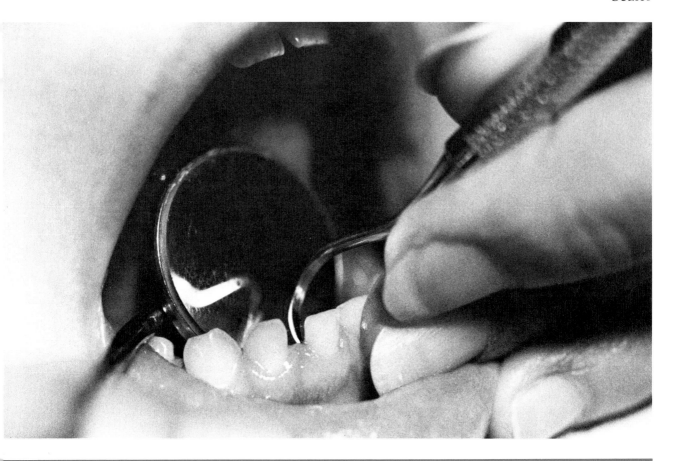

Scaler

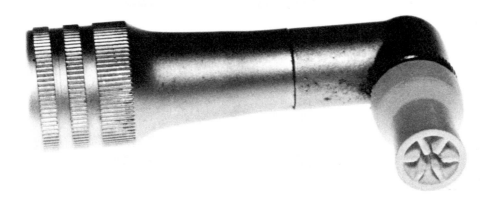

Rubber cup on handpiece

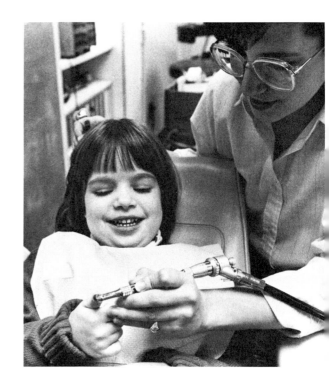

To make sure that every speck of plaque is gone, the hygienist polishes your teeth. The polisher is a tiny **rubber cup.** It is attached to a **handpiece** with a motor that makes the rubber cup spin around. It makes a whirring sound. She may give you

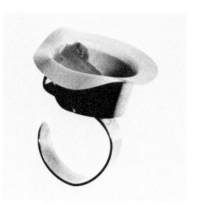

Toothpaste ring

an idea of how it feels by letting it buzz on your thumb. It tickles. It feels the same on your teeth. Paste for the polisher is held in a **toothpaste ring** that is worn on a finger. Or, sometimes, the paste is kept in a little cup on the tray.

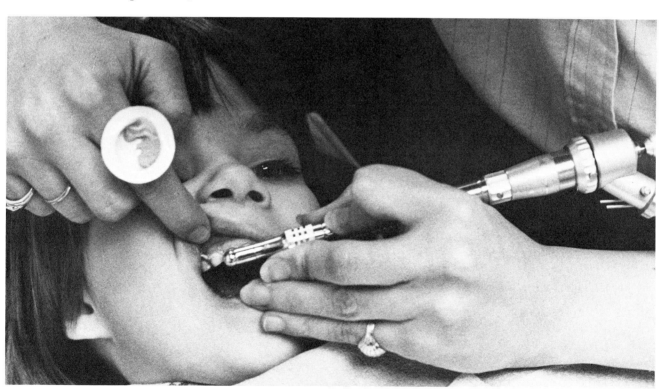

Saliva ejector

When your teeth are being polished, the hygienist uses a **saliva ejector.** It vacuums out the water and leftover paste from your mouth. It makes a bubbly gurgling sound.

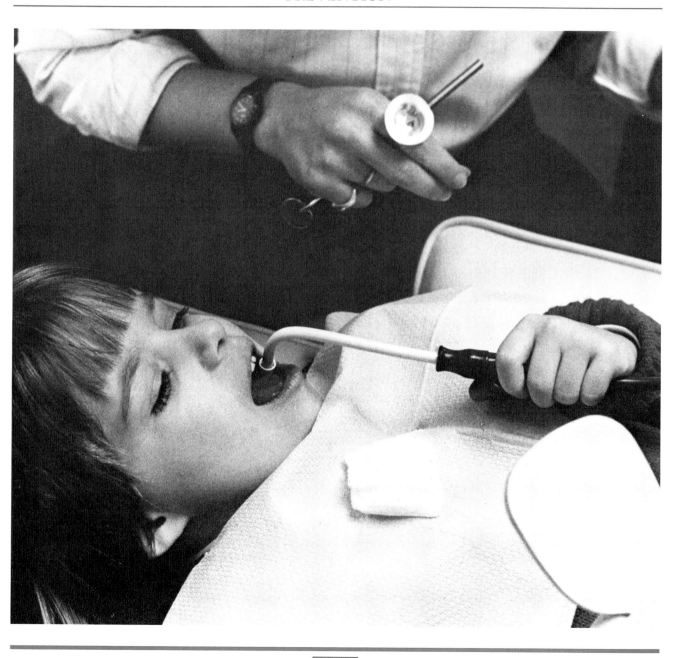

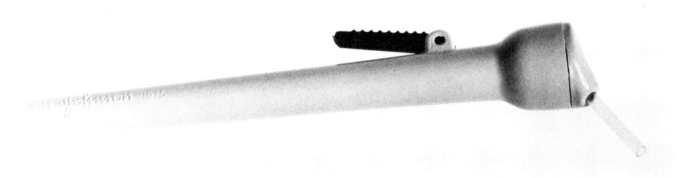

Sealant applicator

Bonding light

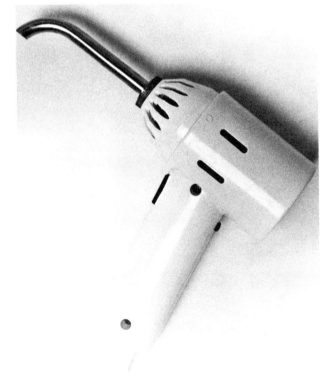

As soon as your teeth are polished, the dentist comes in to check them. If he sees you have a tooth with deep grooves in it, he may want to use a **sealant.** A sealant is a thin layer of strong plastic. It will fill in, or seal up, any natural openings or pits in your tooth that can't be cleaned with a toothbrush. It is put on, drop by drop, with a **sealant applicator.** Some sealants harden by themselves. Others need a special **bonding light** to make them hard. The sealant may make your tooth feel tall. By the next day it will feel fine.

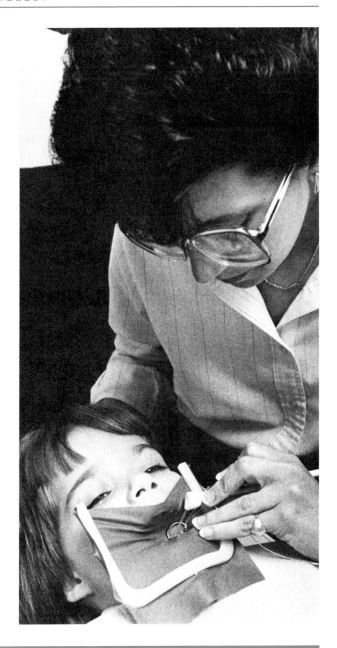

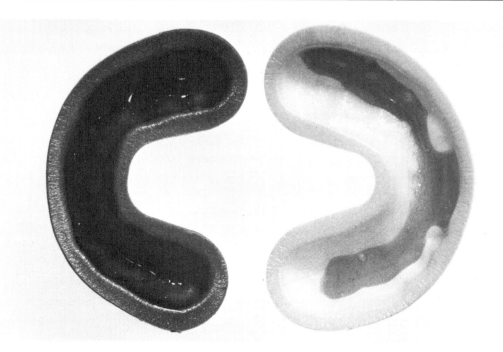

Fluoride tray

The last part of this visit is to have your teeth treated with **fluoride gel** or **paste.** Fluoride is a mineral. It helps make your teeth strong. Sometimes it is painted on your teeth and sometimes it is put in a **fluoride tray** that you bite on for a minute. This kind of fluoride is good for your teeth but not for your stomach, so don't swallow it!

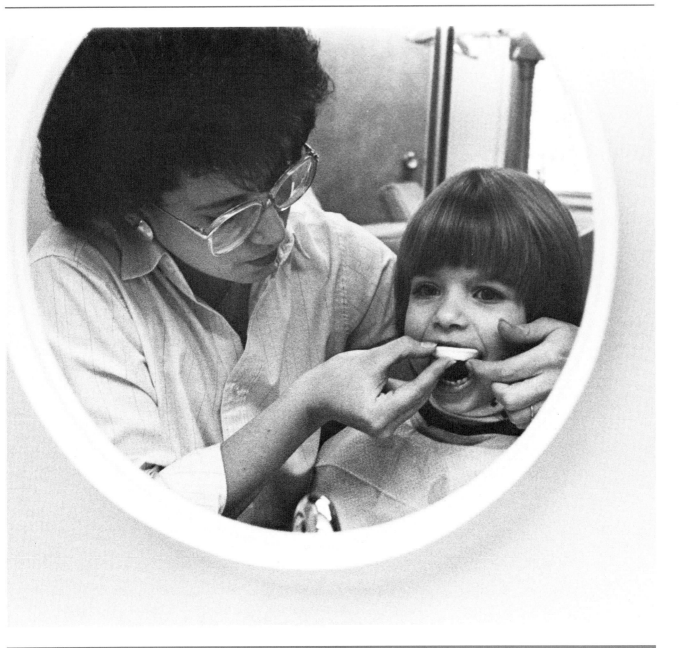

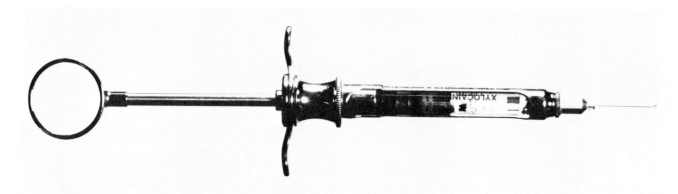

Anesthetic syringe

## REPAIRING A TOOTH

### Filling a Cavity

If your teeth are not brushed and flossed every day, you may get a cavity. A cavity is a hole in your tooth. It is caused by germs in plaque. If it is not fixed, it will get bigger. The dentist's job is to clean out the cavity and put a filling in it. She has special instruments to help her do this.

The dentist uses an **anesthetic syringe** to make your tooth numb. Then it won't hurt while she's fixing it. When she squirts the anesthetic into the gum near your tooth, you might feel a little pinch or a squeeze. It helps if you take some big breaths. Anesthetic doesn't taste good so you will be given some water and told to rinse. Soon your mouth will feel fat and funny. Your tongue and lips may tingle, too. That means the anesthetic from the syringe is working.

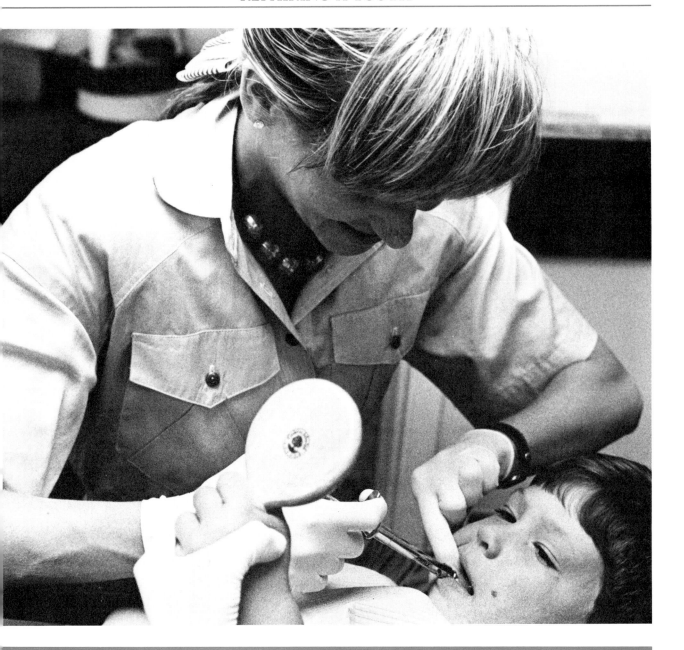

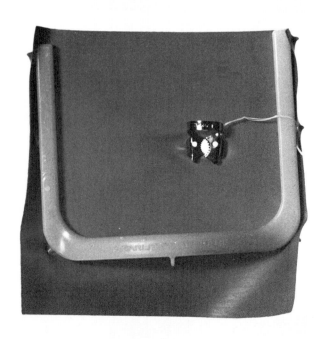

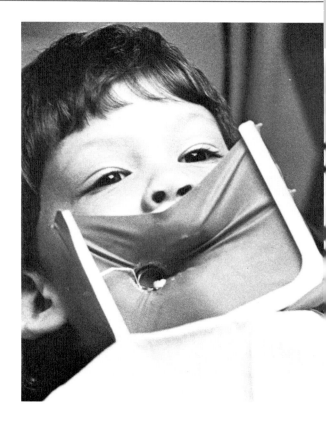

Rubber dam

Some dentists put a **rubber dam** on your mouth before they clean and fill a cavity. It is attached to your tooth with a little buckle. A rubber dam is like a tooth raincoat. It helps your tooth stay dry because your tongue can't bump into it. It also keeps you from having to rinse, spit, and swallow so much.

Three instruments used for cleaning cavities are: a bur, a spoon excavator, and a triplex syringe.

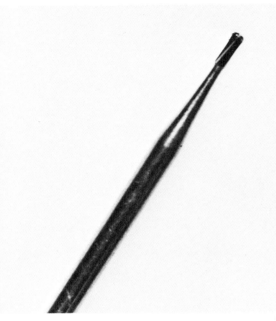

Bur

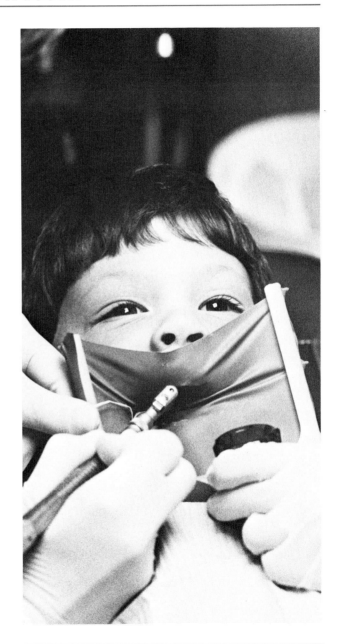

A **bur** is a tiny instrument. It fits on the end of a handpiece. The motor in the handpiece makes the bur whiz round and round. It cleans away the decay from your tooth. At the same time, the handpiece sprays the tooth with cool water. You can feel and hear the bur whizzing, but it doesn't hurt because your tooth is numb.

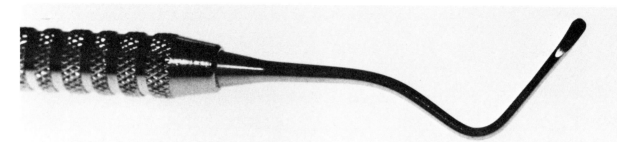

Spoon excavator

The **spoon excavator** is used to scoop out the last bit of decay from the tooth. It makes a scraping sound.

The **triplex syringe** does three things. It squirts water. It sprays water. And it blows air. It is used to wash, rinse, and dry your tooth.

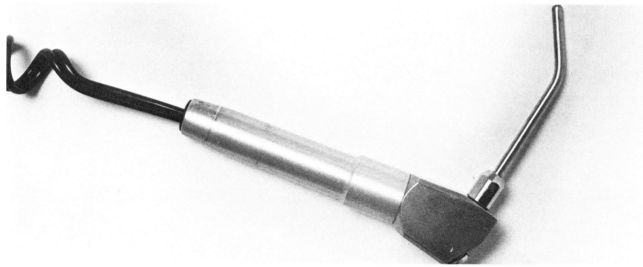

Triplex syringe

After the cavity is cleaned, the dentist may put a **matrix retainer** around your tooth. This little collar will hold the new filling in place.

To keep the cavity dry, the dentist uses big tweezers called **college pliers** to place **cotton rolls** on either side of your tooth. (When you wear a rubber dam she doesn't need to do this.) She also uses the saliva ejector to keep the cavity from getting wet.

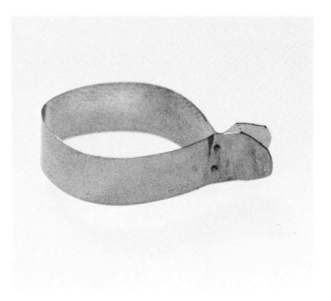

Matrix retainer

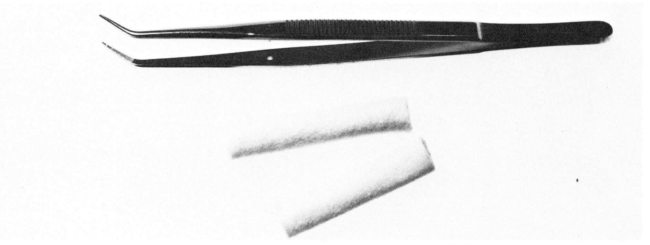

College pliers and cotton rolls

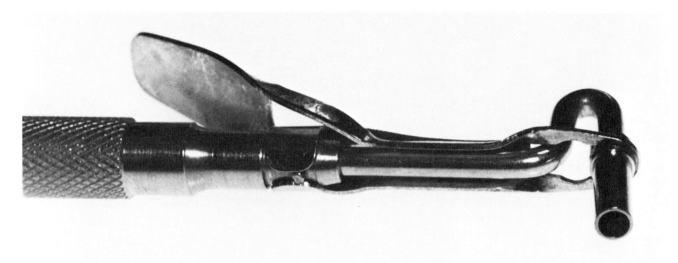

Carrier

There are different instruments for different fillings. For an amalgam or silver filling the dentist uses a carrier, a condenser, a carver, and a burnisher.

The **carrier** picks up the silver and puts it into the cavity. The **condenser** packs it down. The **carver** shapes it, so it won't feel bumpy when you bite down on it. And the **burnisher** rubs it smooth.

For a composite (plastic) filling, the dentist uses a brush, a plastic instrument, a bonding light, and a polishing disc. Plastic fillings are layered onto your teeth.

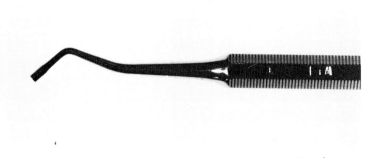

Condenser

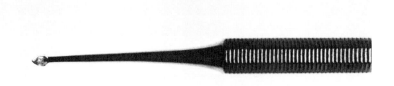

Carver

Burnisher

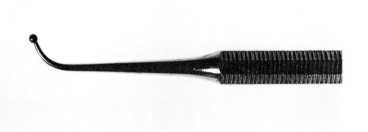

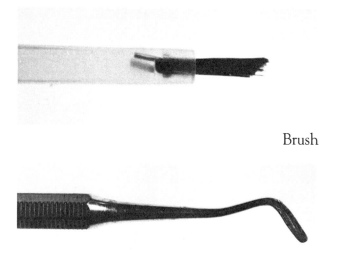

Brush

Plastic instrument

The first layer is brushed on with the **brush tip.** The second is put on with the **plastic instrument.** Both layers are hardened with the **bonding light.** Then, the filling is polished smooth with the **polishing disc.** Unlike silver fillings, plastic fillings are hard to see because they are the same color as your teeth.

It is important to remember that your tooth and mouth will still be numb for a while after your cavity has been filled. So, be careful not to bite or chew on your lips, your tongue, or your cheeks.

Before you go home the dentist may give you a little gift. It might be a balloon, a colored pencil, or maybe even a toothbrush. But the nicest gift she can give you is to help you learn to take the best possible care of your teeth. They are special and so are you.

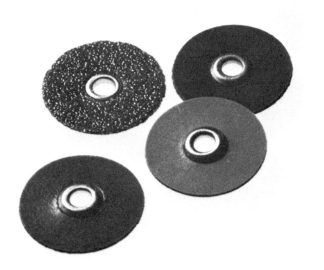

Polishing disc

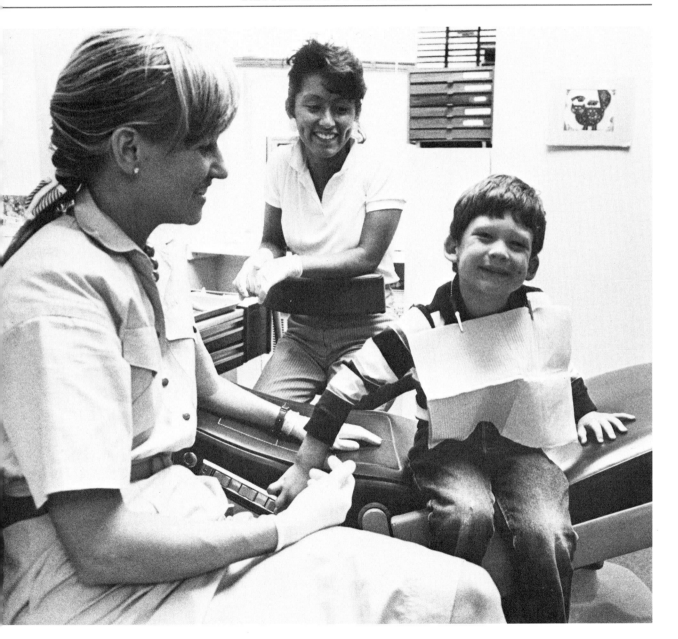